Introduction

The main points

Why bore you with 3000 pages of information, let's face it, you may not remember all that literature, so why confuse you; I have compiled many of the healing practises from around the world, so, I may inform you of their benefits rather than spend all of my time elaborating on inconsumable information which I think is nothing but a story of how someone else did what they did to heal; which I may add, may not work for you, as we are all different and unique in our own ways.

This book is about healing remedies, some you may be aware of and others you may not even heard about.

I talk about what worked in the past; this book is largely to inform people that there are ways that one can heal without buy expensive

medicines. After all medicine came
from somewhere, unless it just
dropped from the sky – it is made
from natural resources of this earth.
The choice is yours; I am only here
to inform you that there are other
ways to heal, however please do not
come off your regular medication
because natural remedies have to be
consumed for a while before the
body can move on to them. Do not
just stop and rely on natural medicine
if you have been on medication from
your doctor.

Think that there are two camps; one camp comprises of medical practitioners' subsequently, the other camp comprises of natural healers, they each have their way of doing things. Going from natural to medical is ok, the body can adapt. However, going from medical to natural can be tricky and can only be done with the consent of your medical practitioner.

Release the tensions, don't worry

<u>For the learner person</u>

Can you do anything about stress?
No

So why worry? Learn from this book.

Can you do anything about stress?
Yes

So why worry? learn more from this
book.

<u>For the clever person</u>

Can you do anything about healing?
No

So why worry? Read this book.

Can you do anything about healing?
Yes

So why worry? Read this book
carefully.

<u>For the common person</u>

Can you do anything about mind
craziness? No

So why worry? follow this book.

Can you do anything about mind
craziness? Yes

So why worry? follow this book
gracefully.

<u>For the teacher person</u>

Can you do anything about the deep
hurt inside? No

So why worry? Teach from this book.

Can you do anything about the deep
hurt inside? Yes

So why worry? Teach and learn from
this book carefully.

<u>For the practitioner's person</u>

Can you do anything about the
confused mind? No

So why worry? practice this book.

Can you do anything about the
confused mind? Yes

So why worry? practise this book and
expand the knowledge.

<u>For the critic's person</u>

Can you do anything about the way
you feel? No

So why worry? exercise this book.

Can you do anything about the way
you feel? Yes

So why worry? observe this book and
remember others are learning too.

<u>For the hater person</u>

Can you do anything about the hatred
that controls you? No

So why worry? Open your mind with
this book.

Can you do anything about the hatred

that controls you? Yes

So why worry? Learn to forgive and

let go.

Chap. 1 – Aromatic healing

The following oils are listed to give some people a brief indication of what they do; and what they can be used for, please consult a herbalist before trying out any of these.

This is mainly because some people have different skin types, this book is here to identify and information about various healing out there and what may work(s) for you.

Every information is here to help you heal if something does not aid in your recovery, please try something else, some professional medical diagnoses patience this way too. But herbal medicine has been around for thousands of years, and none herbal medicine or herbal medicine with is drug-induced for additions or repeat recreation purposes has only been around for a century or more.

Ancient healing oils of aroma

Basil oil –

constipation, healing

diabetes healing

indigestion, healing

motion sickness, healing

nausea, healing

respiratory problems, healing

Bergamot oil –

antibacterial healing

antibiotic properties, healing

digestion healing

infections healing

lower blood pressure healing

pain healing

stress healing

Black pepper oil –

aches healing

antiviral healing

detoxify healing

digestive tonic healing

ease feelings of anxiety healing

pains healing

Camphor oil –

counter irritant healing

eczema healing

helps induce sleep healing

nail fungus healing

pain (on the skin) healing

promotes hair growth healing

swelling (on the surface) healing

treats cold and cough healing

head lice. healing

Chamomile oil –

anti-inflammation healing

anxiety relief healing

arthritis. healing

back pain, healing

eczema healing

gas healing

including ulcers and sores healing

indigestion, healing

nausea, healing

neuralgia, healing

pain healing

promoting sleep healing

rashes. healing

wound healing, healing

Cinnamon oil –

alleviate aches, healing

dry skin, healing

infections. healing

pains, healing

rashes, healing

Clary sage oil –

antibacterial properties healing

antidepressant healing

aromatherapy healing

helps with anxiety healing

menopause symptoms healing

menstrual cramps healing

stress reduction healing

Clove oil –

dental healing

digestive tract, healing

pain, healing

respiratory conditions healing

topical, healing

treating infections, healing

Cocoa butter oil –
fatty acids, healing
hydrate skin healing
improve elasticity healing
natural (phytochemicals) healing
nourish skin healing
protective barrier skin healing

Cyprus oil –
antiseptic
heals infection healing
                                    menstrual
cramps healing
regulate blood flow healing

relieve stress

respiratory system healing

speeds up the healing

Eucalyptus oil –

anti-inflammatory healing

arthritis healing

blocked nose healing

burns healing

cold sores healing

diabetes healing

fever. healing

help lower blood sugar. healing

ulcers. healing

wounds healing

Dit da jow oil –
analgesic liniment healing
improve healing
injuries healing
pain healing
stimulate circulation, healing
swelling, healing
wounds healing

Frankincense oil –
anti-inflammatory healing

anxiety, healing

arthritis healing

improve gut healing

improves asthma healing

joint healing

memory healing

oral health healing

osteoarthritis healing

rheumatoid arthritis healing

                    stress, healing

Geranium oil –
aromatherapy, healing

balances healing

fatigue, healing

hormones healing

improves cognitive purpose, healing

improves concentration, healing

lowers anxiety, healing

lowers emotional strain healing

lowers sadness, healing

lowers stress, healing

lowers tension, healing

Lavender oil –

anti-inflammatory healing

antiseptic healing

depression healing

depression, healing

heal small burns healing

improves minor bug bites healing

helps anxiety, healing

insomnia,

insomnia, healing

restlessness, healing

treating anxiety, healing

Lemon oil –
antifungal healing

antiseptic, healing
astringent, healing
calming, healing
detoxifying, healing
disinfectant healing
energizing healing
stimulating, healing
uplifting scent healing

Lemongrass oil –
acne healing
anxiety healing
aromatherapy healing

bacterial healing

depression healing

fungal healing

headaches healing

insomnia healing

menstrual problems

pain healing

relaxing sore muscles

restlessness healing

stress relief healing

Mandarin oil –
antiseptic

blood healing
bruises healing
digestion healing
pains healing
spasmodic healing
stomach healing
stress healing

Menthol oil –
aesthetic healing
anti-inflammatory, healing
antibacterial, healing
antispasmodic healing

antiviral, healing
carminative healing
discomfort healing
insecticidal, healing

Myrrh oil –
colds, healing
congestions, healing
cough, healing
indigestions healing

                    stomach,
healing

Orange oil –

anticancer healing
antimicrobial healing
antioxidant healing
anxiety healing
aromatherapy healing
depression
depression healing
exercise performance
insecticide healing
pain healing
weight loss healing

Patchouli oil –

anti-inflammatory healing

anti-inflammatory healing

antibacterial healing

antifungal healing

pain healing

weight loss healing

Rosemary oil –

brain healing

bugs repellent healing

circulation healing

hair growth healing

joint healing

pain healing

stress healing

Sandalwood oil –

bronchitis healing

depression healing

fatigue, healing

gallbladder problems, healing

high blood pressure, healing

including anxiety, healing

indigestion, insomnia, healing

low libido, healing

physical and mental disorders,
healing

Tea tree oil –
acne healing
anti-inflammatory healing
antimicrobial healing
calm redness, healing
clear skin healing
inflammation healing
reduce acne scars, healing
smooth, healing
swelling, healing

Thyme oil –
acne healing
cough healing
enhance libido healing
mood, healing
respiratory tract healing

Yiang, Yiang oil –
enhance libido healing
mood, healing
insect repellent, healing

promote wound healing,

inflammation, healing

reduce the appearance of scars,

(apply to skin) healing

                    pain healing

Chap. 2 – Ancient walking healing

Ancient lost walks healing – getting lost and then finding a path of choice. This is based on the concept of finding one's self.

Though losing one's self in an unfamiliar place, a person can start walking the way they feel and not the way they have structured their walk pattern due to the infrastructure of society's conformity of trying to fit in.

Changing the way one walks to fit into
the matrix of culture.

The more we try to fit into the matrix,
the more we distance ourselves from
our individuality. Lost walking
untangles us the person that we are
becoming to the person we are.
Because some of us find ours in a
place where nobody recognizes us, so
we do not need to impress others.

This is also based on Goffman's
concepts of the front stage backstage,

whereby we perform every day for society soon as the curtains open.

However, soon as we are on the backstage, we tend to conform no longer and embrace our individuality. Lost walking brings us the time to find that person inside who is fighting to come out.

Advice: get lost!!!

Backward walking healing – this kind of walking firstly engages the

quadriceps and calves' muscles, which
are not used in the forward walking
motions.

As we use hamstrings and glutes
muscles walking forwards

Secondly, some of us may have a
balance issue, as we do not have eyes
at the back of our heads. So, walking
backward can be tricking. This might
be better practiced in a controlled
environment. And lastly, the mind
unwinds, as the brain has to engage

with the body for this practice to
work.

The more the mind engages its safety
protocol, the less the account will be
focussed on stressful issues, which
have led one to walk backward in the
first place.

Advice: practice now and shed
stress!!!

Bushwalking healing – Indiana Jones
(1981), the golden classics on the

past, introduces a new way to
bushwalk.

Of course, within Indiana Jones, it is
more likely to run from something
rather than walking. We all need a
push of some sort, and a bolder
rolling behind us may give us that bit
of encouragement that some of us
may need time to time.

I mean, some of us need an
adventure to be connected to our day,
so our mind can be connected to

bushwalking in the same way it
engages with social media. Once this
is achieving the possibilist are endless,
and the mind can take a vacation too.

The point I am trying to make is
when some of us find ourselves
bushwalking, we tend to get bored
quickly or distracted with modern-day
technology, which gets in the way of
being with nature.

So, we need that special bolder
behind, which causes us to partake in

the bliss of bushwalking. So next time
adventure walks, bring to light the
Jumanji (2017), the experience of
creating riddles and clues in the brush
so the mind can engage on the here
and now.

Advice: get lost in the bush and create
a way out!!!

Firewalking healing is commonly
known as hot coal walking; it is a
daunting fearful experience before
you burn your feet.

You see, some of us have a narrow
mind of the paranoid, overthinking
view of such experience. We tend to
believe some else's confusing
experience, which may not be
accurate.

Firewalking, is genuinely a mind-
opening experience, imagen all the
fear, paranoia, and the overthinking
mindset suddenly comes to a halt
because our feet have stepped onto

'fire,' it is at that point the mind only focuses on the feet.

The most powerful computer in the world – the mind, stops for them a few moments while we gain an experience of a lifetime. When we come off the fire on the other side, the feeling is unparalleled to any other.

Advice: time to feel the burn!!!

Leisure stroll healing – not a care in the world, well, that's what we want to believe, do we not!!!

Leisurely walking is a must; some of us do not notice when we do this; this may occur on holiday when things are going better than planned, and we get that 'me time' in place.

It is also called slow walking, which of course, is linked to burning more calories because the mind is on vacation, and the muses do not need

to be engaged as per usual with
everyday errands.

Strolling for 2-3 miles also may
reduce the strain on the joints, which
can help with arthritis issues.

Advice: walk slower, take more
considerable strides, and some of us
can limit the walking and lose no
time!!!

The story of the past, the grandfather,
would stroll and further and live

longer, as the youngster walks faster and gets even more now. Still, in the end, the youngster never becomes the grandfather because he walked to fast. So, the grandfather has to walk even slower because he has to push the wheelchair carrying the youngster; the morel is to get there and return; not get to the finish line and respond in a wheelchair.

Lunge walking healing – is an outstanding exercise for establishing a more robust lower body posture. As the legs strengthen your glutes, abs, and hips, will function better as they too become more robust. If you're new to this kind of walking experience, please practice performing a stationed lunge exercise first. As the balance starts to adapt, and the back starts to straighten, we then are ready to move off.

However, the critical part is not to let the knee touch the ground. But bring the knee close to the ground as possible. In the first instance, it is not about how far you go; however, it is how the posture moves.

Because a correct posture will strengthen legs, glutes, abs, and hips, and a bad attitude may have the opposite effect.

As we are here to inform and not an exercise manual, please check out the exercise before attempting anything.

This healing walk brings a feel-good factor into play because this does two things together; we can exercise while walking and strengthening our lower part of our bodies.

Advice: balance and posture control bring great wellness!!!

Prowl walking – prowler uses the walk of the night people, this kind of step, because it keeps them out of sight and gives them the advantage of surprise when they are ready to perform their activities. For the ordinary person, this healing walk brings back the bounce back into their step.

It also pushes and forces the body to move in what may seem like a ridiculous fashion. However, what you are not aware of; is that the prowler uses this walk for a reason, which is that the prowler stimulates and uses all the muscle groups when they do not need to do much.

However, soon as they have been detected, they engage their rested muscles to attempt a getaway.

This works for others, too, to imagine taking the pressure off the muscles, which we use regularly and replace it with muscles we rarely use.

This is why prowler's getaway because they save their energy until they run out of prowler power.

Advice: try it before you shy it away!!!

Somnambulating walking healing is
commonly known as sleepwalking;
The body and mind are trying to
reconnect as the brain is in a
deepened state of sleep. The mind
sometimes transcends with the soul as
the body struggles to cope with its
soul.

Thus, the need for sleep, this is
commonly called astral projection.
The soul and the mind leave during

the night and arrive back when the body has healed.

In some cases, people feel a jolt when walking up. This is because the reconnections process is complete. So, when someone tries to interact with us in the

Somnambulating sleep healing states we tend to be unresponsive. Because we are at that point a zombie and if woken, can stay in that vegetation state.

Next time you see a Somnambulating
sleepwalker healing, please do not
intervene as they are trying to
reconnect with their mind and soul.

Sometimes when the mind and soul
get to the body, they call the
organization to them. It is like a
remote reconnection.

Advice: be mindful of people healing
and try not to intervene!!!

Stride walking healing – walking in long steps can build muscles in the abs, hips, and legs. This is a common belief; however, what is forgotten, that a stride is a distance from where the foot is picked up from and lands.

So the distance from the landed foot to the other foot is the stride. While in the motion of the pace, balance yourself, repeat the process and after every eighteenth stride, stop and check for balance and posture correctness.

And then move off slower than
before, repeat for eighteenth strides,
and recheck the balance and posture
correctness, and this time move even
slower and repeat until you are
moving at the pace of a turtle.

After long, this may strengthen your
hips, legs, glutes, abs, and correct
your posture with your balance,
practice three times a week for
effective results.

Advice: move like a turtle to sore like
an eagle!!!

Stumble walking healing - to miss a
step and stumble in society can be
embarrassing, as the connection of
collectiveness has been interrupted.

The is a glitch in the matrix (Matrix,
1999), it is those glitches we use to
break our bodies out of the matrix of
life's collective walk.

The stubble is usually an indication
that some rest and relation is needed
in one's routine, as the mind is having
trouble connecting with the body. So,
glitches are apparent. Thus, we tend
to fall if the posture and balance are
out too.

There is no sense in walking a tight
rope when a person is exhausted, as it
only can end up in disaster. So,
please heed this warning well; we all
need a time out, and the time out
doesn't mean getting intoxicated, as

that will do nothing other than clouding the mind from connecting. I mean a relaxing and soothing spa with a pamper session that lasts all weekend, if not a day, at least.

Advice: relax it or lose it!!!

Swagger walking healing – this is walking like one has a limp; walk with a lofty proud gait, it is supposed to bring a believer of self-confidence in a person as they bounce or shudder from one step to the next.

The walk comes from animals in the
wild, such as a gorilla, maybe
sometimes an injured gorilla, but a
gorilla.

This is mainly because gorillas are
more durable than most animals, and
when they are angry, they can
become unpredictably ruthless.

So, the swagger walk is connected to
this theory that if a gorilla in the
jungle can do it, so can a youngster in

the hood. Of course, without the power and sheer brute force of a gorilla's might.

Advice: animals walk, humans copy!!!

Tai chi walking – this walk is known as the correct walk in the martial arts domain. As it is believed, a person must stand upright, and they must lean into their step, as did Indi (Harrison ford) in Indiana Jones in the last crusade (1989) when he leaped faith. And soon after one

lands, the waist must shudder left and
then right, forcing the hip to bring the
back leg forward.

This helps in one of two ways, the
first helps keep balance, as you can
see in the film of Indiana Jones in the
last crusade (1989); the second is
posture control if done correctly.
However, to do this successfully, we
must loosen the waist.

And become like the willow tree,
because the willow tree is through to

stay intact, even in a gale-force wind
due to its flexibility. Flexibility being
the keyword, the more flexible one is
the posture and balance with aid its
path.

Advice: walk of faith, for each step in
unknown!!!

Trudge walking healing is strolling as
the feet are plugged firmly into the
next step. Such as weary, or through
the mud. I remember once when we

were on an archaeology field trip, we were hiking and we came across a muddy field, it was surely an experience walking in knee height mud.

But from my experience, I learned that each time I dragged my foot out of the mud to take another step, I could feel my hamstrings, calves, and glutes engaged.

Instead of dragging pulling and struggling, I started to walk like a giant, and to my surprise, my legs got stronger that day. I think the day was the day I decided to practice different walks to build my legs stronger.

Advice: unleash the giant step and seek the rewards!!!

Wave walking healing – this comprises of walking through water, please practice this in a swimming pool before trying it in the ocean.

This walk, I was taught by my aqua aerobics' instructor. I was surprised; the more I walked forward faster, the more I struggled to keep balance.

The additional resistance allows one to challenge, intensify, and strengthen the muscles. It also helps one burn calories, help in weight loss, and it will loosen stiff muscles, which have hardened through life's stressful challenges.

This water exercise helps reduce
stress levels if done in the sea due to
the sea being rich in minerals and
salt.

Advice: wave the calories and stress
away!!!

Side walking healing – side shifting
walking routine is mainly an exercise
unless you would like to walk
sideways. It works the glutes to
perform a pumped like booty; a
round posterior is you wish. It also

works the hamstrings and engages the
side muscles, which we do not use
much. Please be careful as stumbling
may happen because it is abnormal
for some of us to walk in this manner.

Advice: sidestep to the left, sidestep
to the right!!!

Staggered walking – ok, ok, I know
what you are thinking, and you are
right, it is the drunken sail walk. It is
commonly performed when

intoxicated due to the staggered-ness of the individual.

This walk is happening not only because the person does not have coordination; it is also because we are walking without thinking about where our next step goes. In our ruffled and disorientated state, we tend to behave erratically and unpredictably. And not to mention, we tend to talk to ourselves as we no longer conform to the boundaries of society, well until someone witnesses or sees us.

This may ease the mind and move
the posture in ways you didn't think
you had in you because, for a brief
period, you become the willow tree
which now can flow in any direction
until the morning when the elixir of
the night before has faded in one's
system.

Advice: let go, and stagger away!!!

Wind swaying walking – this is
walking in a heavy gale-force like

wind, it is near impossible to push the leg out, let alone walk. So, what do I do here, this walk may help some. Learn forward like the moonwalk from Michael Jackson and try and balance before taking the first step, let the wind hold you and then move by jolting the hip forward as a salsa dancer would.

We dance the Mexican dance of the Salsa to the gale's music and to whatever song we like, as long as we move in the salsa way, the wind

simply moves through us rather than
against us.

Advice: move like the wind, and Salsa
will be the guide!!!

Chap. 3 – Healing powders and talc's

Alum powder –

May have antiseptic properties

May assist with reducing bleeding

May help with minor abrasions

May assist with cuts

May assist nosebleeds

Many more benefits of using these powders and talcs...

Just may assist; just may not assists;
however, if you don't try, you may
never know what works and what
doesn't.

Amway persona talc –

May assist with sweat absorption
May reduce body smell
May have a cooling effect.

Many more benefits of using these
powders and talc's...

Just may assist; just may not assists; however, if you don't try, you may never know what works and what doesn't.

Antiseptic body powder –

May have antiseptic properties.

Many more benefits of using these powders and talc's...

Just may assist; just may not assists;
however, if you don't try, you may
never know what works and what
doesn't.

Baby powder –

May have antiseptic properties
May avert from diaper rash
May treat diaper rash
May assist with genital odours (adults)
May help soothing rashes (adults)
May alleviate from friction
May help with genital odours (adults)

May help soothing rashes (adults)
May alleviate friction.

Many more benefits of using these
powders and talc's...

Just may assist; just may not assists;
however, if you don't try, you may
never know what works and what
doesn't.

Boroplus prickly heat talc –

May alleviate from prickly heat

May prevent heat rash

May prevent minor skin infections

May assist with sweat absorption

May reduce body smell

May have a cooling effect that keeps

one fresh.

Many more benefits of using these

powders and talc's...

Just may assist; just may not assists;

however, if you don't try, you may

never know what works and what
doesn't.

Cuticura body powder –

May assist with heat rash
May help with itching sensations
May help with prickly heat
May assist with bacteriostatic issues
May help with sweat absorption
May have a cooling effect
May assist with chaffing
May assist with rubbing
May help with soothing skin

May assist with eczema.

Many more benefits of using these
powders and talc's...

Just may assist; just may not assists;
however, if you don't try, you may
never know what works and what
doesn't.

Demi fresh body heat powder –

May assist with heat rash
May help with itching sensations

May help with prickly heat
May assist with bacteriostatic issues
May help with sweat absorption
May have a cooling effect.

Many more benefits of using these
powders and talc's...

Just may assist; just may not assists;
however, if you don't try, you may
never know what works and what
doesn't.

Gokul Santol body powder –

May add brightness to one's skin

May reduce body smell

May have a cooling effect

May assist even texture to one's skin.

Many more benefits of using these

powders and talc's...

Just may assist; just may not assists;

however, if you don't try, you may

never know what works and what

doesn't.

Clotrimazole body powder –

May have antiseptic properties

May assist with sweat absorption

May reduce body smell

May have a cooling effect

May assist with antifungal

May help with itching sensations

May help with jock itch

May assist with bacteriostatic issues

May assist with ringworm.

Many more benefits of using these
powders and talc's...

Just may assist; just may not assists;
however, if you don't try, you may
never know what works and what
doesn't.

Lavender talc –

May assist with eczema
May have antiseptic properties
May assist with chafing
May help with dry skin
May assist thicken eyelashes
May help with smooth legs

May have a cooling effect

May decrease stress

May assist with itching sensations.

Many more benefits of using these powders and talc's...

Just may assist; just may not assists; however, if you don't try, you may never know what works and what doesn't.

Medipure body powder –

May assist with heat rash

May help with itching sensations

May help with prickly heat

May help with sweat absorption

May have a cooling effect

May assist with chaffing

May assist with rubbing

May assist with soothing skin.

Many more benefits of using these
powders and talc's...

Just may assist; just may not assists;
however, if you don't try, you may

never know what works and what
doesn't.

Modern medical body powder –

May assist with heat rash
May help with itching sensations
May help with prickly heat
May help with sweat absorption
May have a cooling effect
May assist with chaffing
May assist with rubbing
May help with soothing skin

May assist with burning

May assist with crackling

May assist jock itch

May help with athletes' foot

May assist ringworm

Many more benefits of using these

powders and talc's...

Just may assist; just may not assists;

however, if you don't try, you may

never know what works and what

doesn't.

Navigating body powder –

May assist with heat rash

May help with itching sensations

May help with prickly heat

May help with sweat absorption

May have a cooling effect

May assist with chaffing

May assist with rubbing

May assist with soothing skin.

Many more benefits of using these
powders and talc's...

Just may assist; just may not assists;
however, if you don't try, you may
never know what works and what
doesn't.

Shower powder – shower to shower

May assist with breathing
May assist with brain functions
May assist nervous systems
May assist with muscles
May help with sweat absorption
May have a cooling effect.

Many more benefits of using these powders and talc's...

Just may assist; just may not assists; however, if you don't try, you may never know what works and what doesn't.

Summer body powder –

May assist with sweat absorption
May reduce body smell
May reduce irritation

Many more benefits of using these powders and talc's...

Just may assist; just may not assists; however, if you don't try, you may never know what works and what doesn't.

Chap. 4 – Ancient abandoned healing

A scare – for hiccups

Acai – multi health purposes

Almonds – multi health purposes

Aloe – for burns

Apples – multi health purposes

Avocados – for papercuts and burns

Beans – multi health purposes

Blackberries – for diarrhoea

Blueberries – multi health purposes

Brandy – dabbed on tooth pain
surrounding

Buttermilk – for age spots

Capsaicin – for psoriasis

cherries – for gout

Chia seeds – multi health purposes

Chicken soup – for flu and colds

Clove – for tooth pain

Coke a cola & milk mix – for stress

Cold tea bags – for puffy eyes

Cranberry juice(s) – for UTI's

Cucumber – for eye strain

Dark chocolate – for weight loss

Dates & Figs – are award-winning as
outstanding sources of energy when
ill.

Egg-yolk – build an immune system
when ill.

Eucalyptus oil – for runny nose and
sinusitis issues

Fennel – for indigestion

Fenugreek seeds – multi health
purposes

Gee – is a rejuvenating and longevity-
promoting food.

Gəʊbi – for heartburn

Ginger tea – for nausea

God liver and Omega 3 oil –
inflammation –

100

Green tea – for joint pains

Ground flaxseed – for constipation

Honey – ingestion burn –

Horehound tea – for sore throat

Lassi – improves, bones, promotes,
youthful skin, prevents bloating,
immune system, and digestion.

Lavender – for foot smell.

Lemon – for motion sickness.

Lucozade (original) and honey – fever
and aches

Milk of magnesium – for sores

Mung beans – supress hunger

Niacin – for high cholesterol

Olive oil – for cracked lip –

Olives – for blurred vision, vitamin E

peppermint oil – for headaches

Racquets ball – for achy feet

Sage – for memory loss

Sea salt – for yeast infections.

Seawater – for sores

Soy – for osteoporosis

Stress balls – for stress

Sugar – for hiccups

Tea tree – for foist

Thyme tea – for coughs

Turmeric – multi health purposes

Valerian – for insomnia

Vaseline - for small cuts, (boxing federations around the world still use this)

Vitamin A – for younger skin

Warm oil on the forehead – alleviate stress.

Wet cold towel – for headaches

Witches hazel – haemorrhoids

Chap. 5 – Foods that are there for you

Here are a few which we have tried and got health benefits from; some of us result to eating what we desire due to the uncontrollable desires to follow our smell beacon of radar. But when health problems come, some of us, focus of a healthier lifestyle so we can keep in better health as we grow older. So those of you who have reached the health regime, please

take a look below, and those who
haven't quite got there yet, please
come back and read below when the
time is right for you.

Carrots – great source of fibre,
vitamin K1, beta carotene, and
potassium.

Corn – great source of vitamin B12,
iron, lowers cholesterol level and
blood sugar.

Garlic – great source of manganese, vitamin B6, and C, Selenium and Fibre.

Grapefruit – great source of protein, magnesium, thiamine, potassium, vitamin, A and C, fibre, folate and carbs.

Hazelnuts – great source of calcium, vitamins B and E.

Kale – great source of antioxidants, vitamin K and C, calcium, and fibre.

Kiwi - great source of vitamin C, K,
E, folate, antioxidants and potassium.

Mango - great source of protein,
vitamin, C, folate and copper.

Mushrooms - great source of iron,
potassium, cobalamin, vitamin B6, C,
D, and Calcium.

Oats - great source of phosphorus,
magnesium, copper, vitamin B1,
selenium, and iron.

Oats milk- great source of protein, vitamin B12, riboflavin, and calcium.

Onions - great source of vitamin B6, C, magnesium, fibre, potassium, and iron.

Oranges - great source of vitamin A, C, calcium, and magnesium.

Oregano - great source of phytonutrients, antioxidants, iron, tryptophan, vitamin E, K, and fibre.

Peanuts – great source of vitamin B6,
E, magnesium, iron, phosphorous,
copper, potassium, zinc, selenium
and manganese.

Pears – great source of protein, carbs,
fibre, vitamin C, K, potassium and
copper.

Pistachios – great source of
carbohydrates, potassium,
magnesium, and protein.

Porridge – great source of
phosphorus, magnesium, copper,
vitamin B1, selenium, zinc, and iron.

Potato's – great source of vitamin B6,
E, phosphorous, potassium,
magnesium, and copper.

Prawns – great source of vitamin A,
B12, B6, E of calcium, phosphorous,
niacin, and potassium,

Salmon – great source of omega-3,
vitamins A. C, B6, B12, magnesium,
minerals, protein, potassium, and
selenium.

Sesame – great source of vitamin B6,
E, zinc, selenium, copper, and iron.

Spinach – great source of vitamins A,
E, potassium, magnesium, iron,
calcium, and protein.

Strawberries – great source of
vitamins A, E, phosphorous,

potassium, magnesium, iron, calcium,
fibre and protein.

Sunflower seeds – great source of
vitamins E, potassium, magnesium,
copper, and selenium.

Watermelon – great source of
vitamins A, B6, C, magnesium, iron,
lycopene,
 and amino acids and antioxidants.

Yogurt – great source of vitamins
B12, potassium, phosphorous,
calcium, magnesium, iron, calcium,
riboflavin, and protein.

Chap. 6 – Ancient Yoga – the different types

Vinyasa – Vinyasa, similarly also called "flow yoga" due to the way that the poses connect, Vinyasa yoga is the most practiced classification around because it incorporates different yoga techniques into one form.

What health benefits are there from
Vinyasa yoga:

Stability,

Balance,

Power,

Combat anxiety issues,

Relax the mind form high-stress
levels,

Improved cardio,

Muscular physic,

Fitness level upgrade,

What health benefits are there from
Vinyasa yoga:

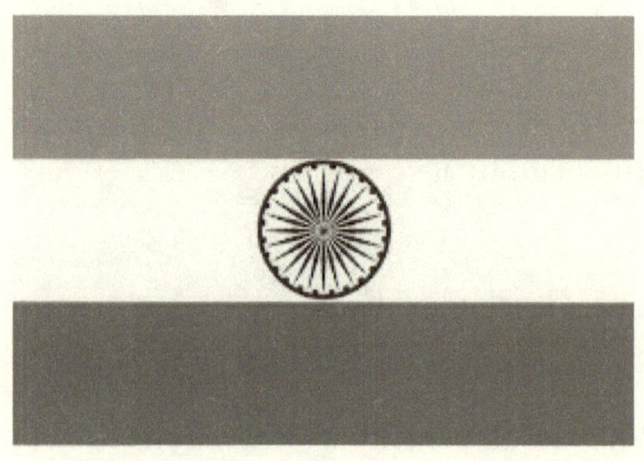

Ashtanga – is a muscular flow yoga that conjoins litheness power and endurance in its practice. Ashtanga yoga's health benefits are to access one's inner peace and be one with the earth, which also aids with stress management. This type of yoga will help in the personnel growth of a person by strengthening the individual from the inside out. Although to achieve this, there are five possess that need to be mastered before the body can become one with the universe and heal.

What health benefits are there from
Ashtanga yoga:

Muscular physic,

Fitness level upgrade,

Mental focus,

Balance coordination,

Spiritual healing and wellness,

Strengthens physicality issues,

Retrains the mind for the inner piece,

Improved cardio,

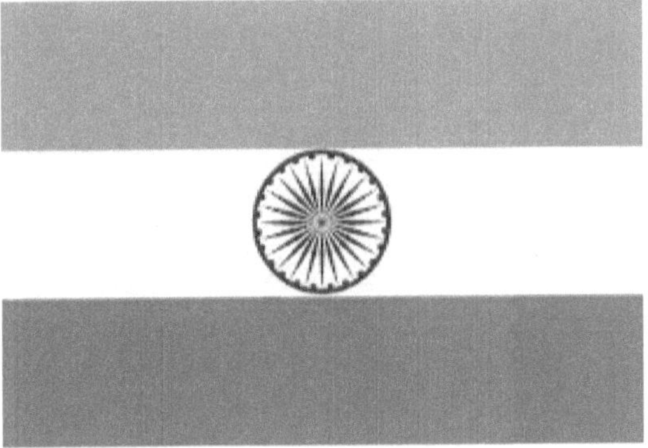

Ashtanga yoga originates from
Mysore, India (1948).

Iyengar – is a Yoga that structurally aligns the physical body; this is carried out by the practice of asanas. Iyengar is different from other types of yoga. It mainly focuses on precision and sequence in which the moves are performed, and within the yoga, exercise props are used to align the body in asana technique. The accessories are used to support and aid the body further into a pose so that the body can extend its stretching capabilities.

What health benefits are there from
Iyengar yoga:

Muscular physic,

Mental focus,

Retrains the mind for the inner piece,

Increase one's flexibility,

Tone muscles and posture,

Pain relief,

Improved breathing,

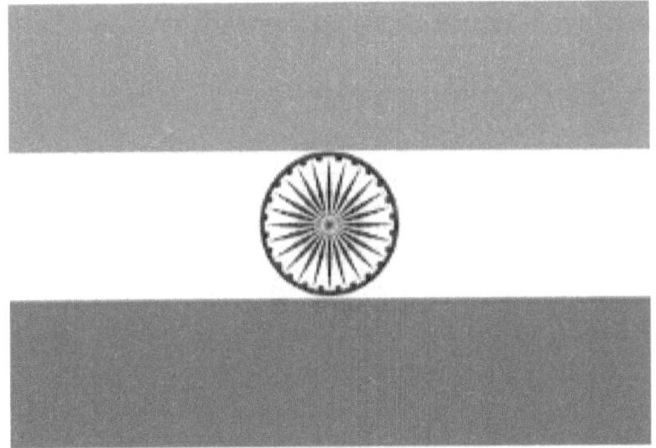

Iyengar yoga originates from India (1936).

Bikram – this type of yoga is usually done in a heated room or exceeding the body temperature gauge. The practice includes repeatedly repeating the same poses to engage the mules and gain a more robust posture while the excess body fat leaves the body due to muscles toning themselves.

What health benefits are there from Bikram yoga:

Tone muscles and posture,

Pain relief,

Promotes weight loss,

Energize,

Fitness level upgrade,

Spiritual healing and wellness,

Retrains the mind for the inner piece,

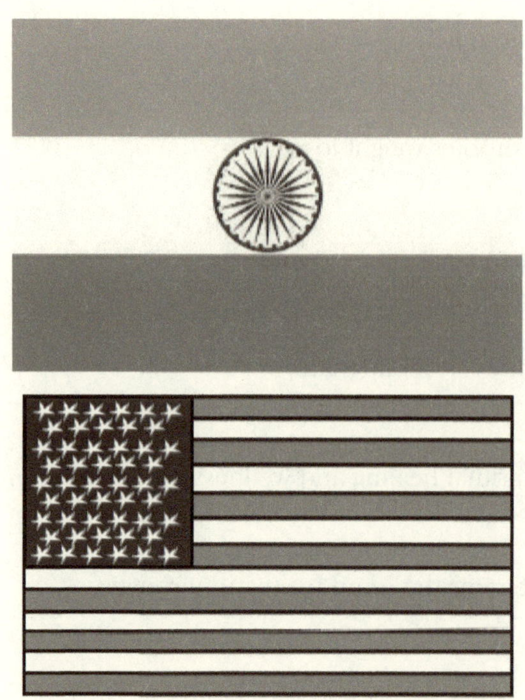

Bikram yoga originates from India and then moved to the united states of American (1970's).

Power – Power yoga integrates the suppleness of Ashtanga yoga, including parts of vinyasas. With its prominence on flexibility and strength-based poses and exercises, power yoga transported yoga into public gyms, which allowed people to experience the real art of healing. Power yoga enhances posture control, stamina, strength, mental focus, and flexibility. It relieves symptoms of tension and releases any toxins through sweat during exercise. It also burns far more calories than any traditional form; therefore, it can promote weight loss.

What health benefits are there from Power yoga:

Relax the mind form high-stress levels,

Improved cardio,

Muscular physic,

Fitness level upgrade,

Muscular physic,

Tone muscles and posture,

Pain relief,

Improved breathing,

Tone muscles and posture,

Promotes weight loss,

Retrains the mind for the inner piece,

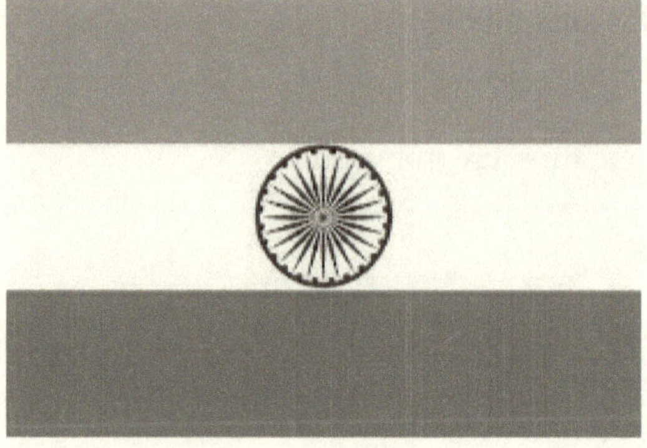

Power yoga originates from Ashtanga Vinyasa Yoga, which gave rise to various styles of yoga as spinoff's, it dates back to 1990's.

Sivananda – this method of yoga is to promote physical healing, which mentally exercises the spiritual wellness of the individuals. The Sivananda system is complexed and needs to be followed through as a set exercise routine. Slow and precise moves are required to do this type of

yoga, and emphasis on detail is
essential because of the spiritual
factors which come together to aid in
the corrective-ness of healing. In
India, the philosophy is surrounding
Sivananda yoga is that it brings
excellent wellness and wellbeing to a
person through the enlightenment of
the enslaved body within. Sivananda
yoga is a healing system like no other,
as it is designed to maintain a healthy
state through spirituality.

What health benefits are there from

Sivananda yoga:

Fitness level upgrade,

Spiritual healing and wellness,

Retrains the mind for the inner piece,

Mental focus,

Increase one's flexibility,

Improved breathing,

Positive and optimistic healing,

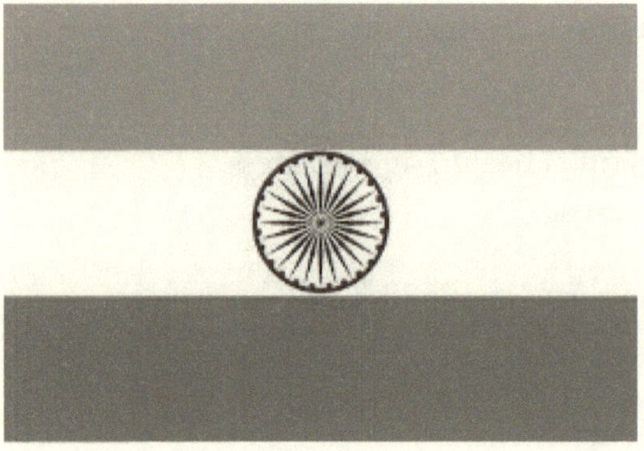

Sivananda yoga originates from
Kerala, south India (1957).

Yin – this type of yoga is from the traditional Taoist monks who have linked the movements to heal. Due to repetitive movements of the body, which creates forces the body to overheat, which then pushes the body to its extremes by being still for more extended periods in the poses, which are partaken in. Yin movements and postures are about finding complete stillness of the body. The moment as the body cools, that is the moment the exercise has reached its climax state.

What health benefits are there from
Yin yoga:

Experience a calmness of energy and
unblocking the flow of energy,

Improves anxiety issues,

Reduces stress,

Circulatory system benefits,

Increases joints mobility.

Increases one's flexibility,

Spiritual healing and wellness,

Balances the internal organs,

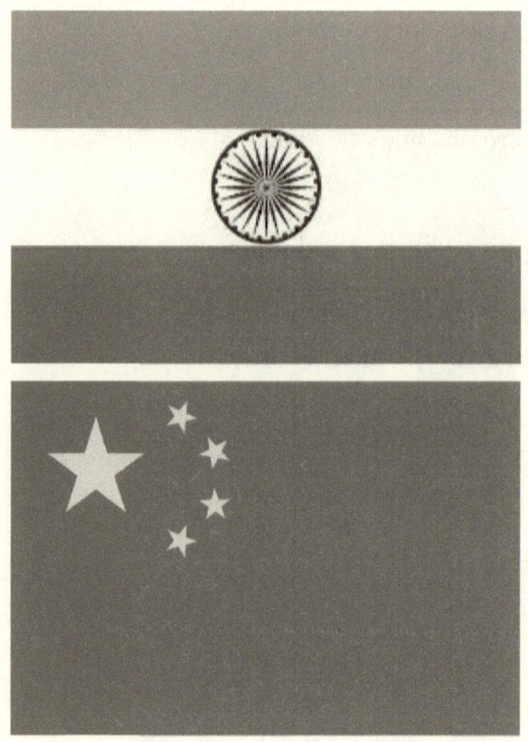

141

Yin yoga originates from India and then went to China (1970's).

Hatha – this is a method of yoga that includes a few yoga styles of other yoga's. It is one of the eldest's systems incorporating the traditional form of asanas yoga (yoga movements through postures). Hatha yoga includes pranayama (deep breathing techniques), which bring the body, mind, and soul into a more profound spiritual status, similar to that of meditation.

What health benefits are there from
Hatha yoga:

Promotes weight loss,

Strengthens the core,

Makes skin feel better,

Immune system benefits,

Heart finality improves,

Align the spine,

Gain tighter his,

Tone muscles and posture,

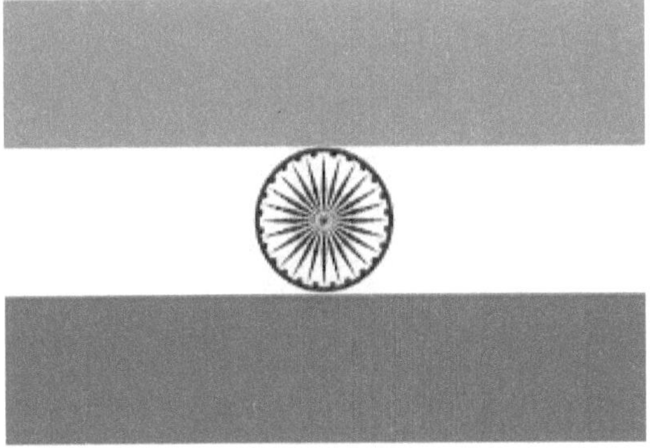

144

Hatha yoga originates from India (it dates back to the 9th century).

Kundalini - awakens is a particular
type of yoga that opens the mind
through spiritually challenging the
mind while engaging in slow yoga
movements. Kundalini yoga increases
brain activity and can adapt the brain
functions to work better, as we are in
the middle of the social media era.
Kundalini yoga can be seen as
therapy of the intellectual mind that
works to ease the daily tensions of
continuous media onslaught,
interaction, and collective pressure.

What health benefits are there from
Kundalini yoga:

Fitness level upgrade,

Spiritual healing and wellness,

Improved breathing,

Positive and optimistic healing,

Reduces stress,

Strengthens your nervous system,

Gain inner peace,

awakened mind,

increases intuition,

increases one's willpower,

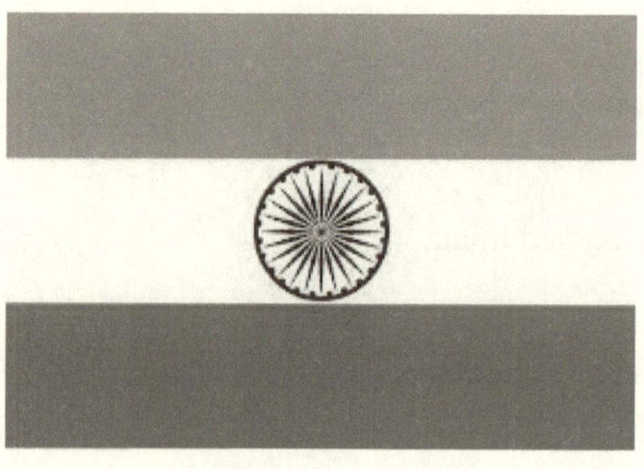

Kundalini yoga originates from India
and brought to the west (1969).

Restorative – this yoga is an excellent
way to separate one from the chaotic
pursuit(s), of daily life and reset your
mind balance meter. Restorative yoga
offers a mind and body alliterating
experience through deepened
meditation awareness. Through slow
moments one gains solidarity of mind
during pose(s) shifting, allowing one
to explore the heightened state of
your mind through a mixture of
balanced and physical tempo
movements. One of spiritual
restorative yoga's shortened names is

"mindful yoga" because it expands
consciousness by making the mind
aware of other possibilities of healing.

What health benefits are there from
Restorative yoga:

Heals emotional anxiety issues,

Improves sleeping,

Improved breathing,

Illness recovery,

Reduces stress,

Strengthens your nervous system,

Gain inner peace,

awakened mind,

increases intuition,

weight loss,

Helps with pain,

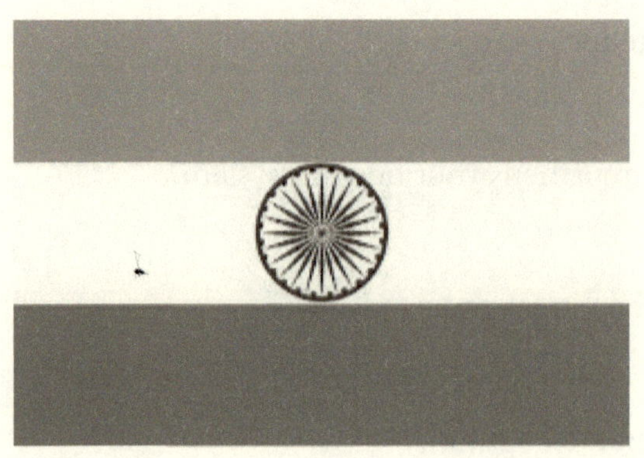

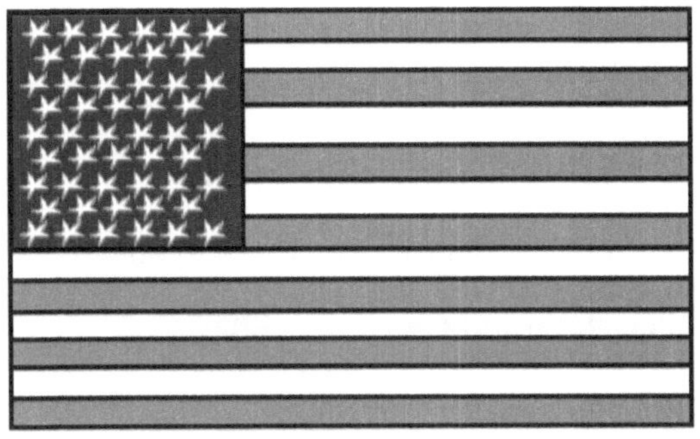

Restorative yoga originates from India based on the fundamental principles of other yoga's techniques and then it has been brought across to the western world.

Prenatal – this type of yoga haves a unique seating status, such as sitting cross-legged because the energy is activated through the chakras through which the mind can gain solidarity. This exercise is mainly conducted on mats prearranged in a circle; this type of yoga is also maidly done by females who are with children. This type of yoga gives the kind of experience of having underwater expertise, which helps the mind relax due to the women being in their second and third trimesters of

pregnancies. Prenatal helps
strengthen the mind-body and spirit
to prepare the women for giving
birth.

What health benefits are there from
Prenatal yoga:

Heals with lower back pain,

Improves sleeping,

Improved strength,

156

Improved suppleness,

Improves breathing,

Decreases lower back pain,

Decreases nausea,

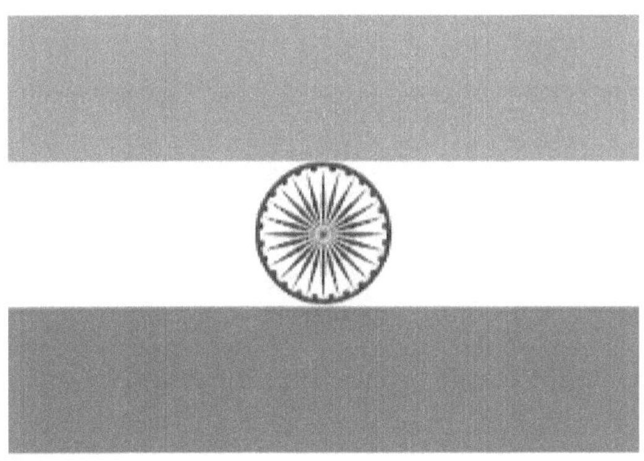

Prenatal yoga originates from the
west, but it is based on the concepts
of yoga from India (2005).

Anusara – after a class of this type of yoga, you'll feel rejuvenated like never before, including increased suppleness, strength, and deep inner peace. Anusara yoga offers a profound focus on aligning the body balance with its chakras, mainly through the five elementary ideologies: when beginning the yoga practice (s), inner spiral, outer spiral, strength-based energy, and prana or chi energy.

What health benefits are there from Anusara yoga:

Heals with lower back pain,

Improves sleeping,

Improved flexibility,

Tone muscles and posture,

Increases joints mobility,

Posture control,

Strengthens tendons,

Healthier lifestyle,

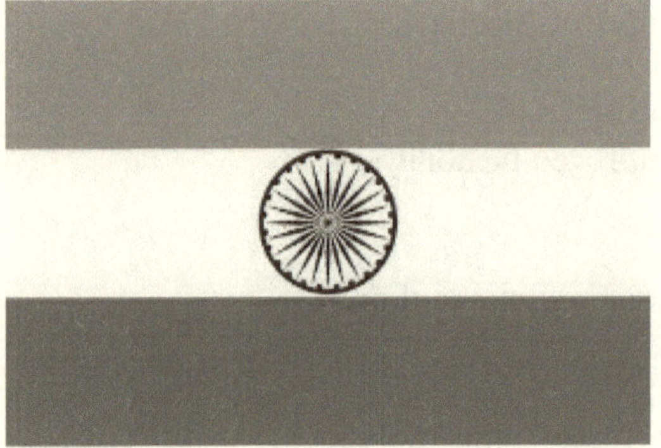

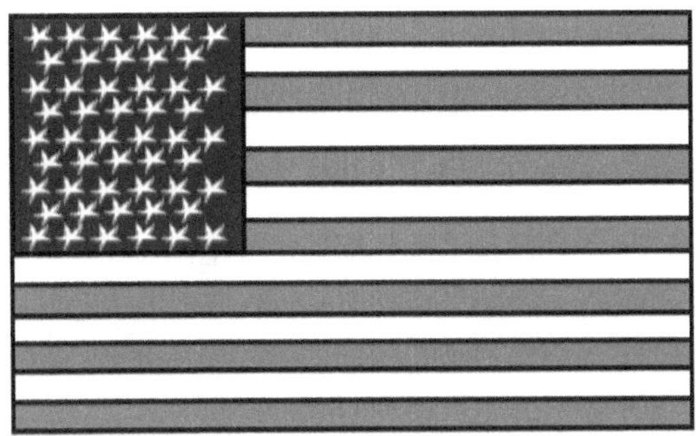

Anusara yoga originates from India, and then moved to the united states of America (1997).

Jiuamukti – the substantial rewards
from this type of yoga include
increased strength, wellness, extra
energy, balance, and suppleness.

Jiuamukti boosts of having high
detoxifying capabilities for improving
the body circulation system, including
a decreased state of stress and body
toxins. Spiritual healing of this yoga
includes self-discovery and the
awareness of oneness, basically how
to be happy alone. Yoga practice(s)
cultivates the one inside by

ascertaining an uninterrupted pranic

joining to the source of blissfulness –

The divine driver within.

What health benefits are there from

Jiuamukti yoga:

Improves body balance,

Improved breathing,

Improved flexibility,

Tone muscles and posture,

Improves circulation,

Detoxifies the body,

Promotes strength increase,

Balances the body dynamics,

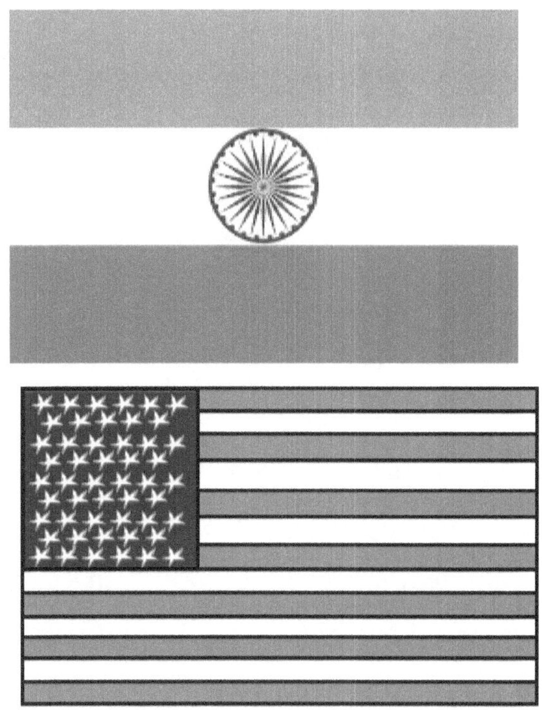

Jiuamukti yoga originates from Manhattan, New York, United States of America (1984).

Pranayama – this type of yoga should be practiced daily because it alleviates the mind from stress and the daily incantations the brain has to perform; it further induces the mind into a meditative state(s). Hypertension, pressure, and high anxiety issues are suppressed, and diminished whist's in this state of meditative yoga.

Pranayama yoga helps to condense frustrating behaviour(s).

Anger, and snappy uncontrollable
issues that are in auto-response to
autosuggestions of the mind due to
irritability

Through channelling energy through
a panoply of breathing exercises, the
person can calm the mind and the
screaming inner child.

Pranayama yoga brings new insight to
the practice of breath, and some say it
is the heart of yoga practice

What health benefits are there from

Pranayama yoga:

Improved flexibility,

Improves breathing,

Improves body balance,

Improves circulation,

Detoxifies the body,

Improves sleeping,

169

Healthier lifestyle,

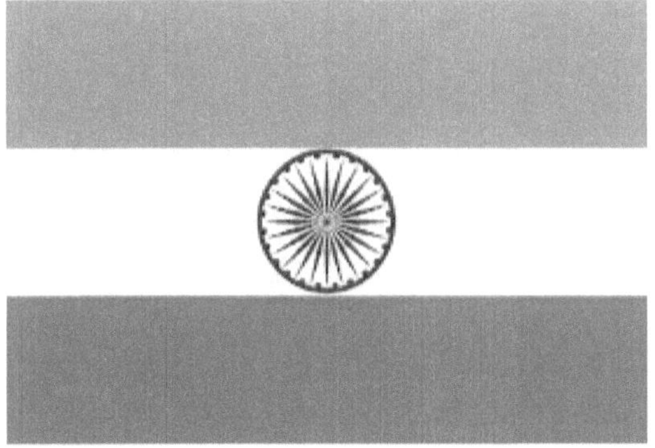

Pranayama yoga originates from
ancient India (fifth and sixth BCE).

Chap. 7 – Description healing

1.   Get rid of pity parties inside the head.

2.   Clear anxious thoughts by thinking that you have a hoover in your head, suck them out.

3.   Challenge yourself doubt.

4.   Tell yourself to set a particular time to worry about general things.

5.   Diminish rumination of stress, as this only magnifies the issues and problems, focus on problem-solving.

6.   Focus on the inner mental muscles that need a gym workout (meditation).

7.   Switch off and do some yoga.
However, you may want to look at the
Yoga section of this book to identify
which yoga you require.

8.   Try guided hypnosis, which
can be found on YouTube for free,
relaxing that heavy daily traffic in the
mind.

9.   Get a balanced sleep, which is
8 hours for an adult, but if you have a
stressful job, you may require more.

10.   Time your sleep means the timing is critical as 10 pm should be the last hour of walk-fullness—however, 8 pm for our small people.

11.   Sleep imbalances – a shower before bed, to warm up the mid ready for a good night or a relaxing bubble bath with candles.

12.   Sexual healing - this can relax
two people and make a good night
sleep more bliss for both

13.   Read a book, as knowledge is
the key to the world, so start reading
something new.

14.   Learn new recipes and cook –
some people use this as stress
therapy, as it helps speed up the
thinking patterns and then slow them
down as you come to a final decision.

15.	Clean up; this can go hand in hand with clearing the thoughts out of one's mind; think each thing you clean, your brain has one less thing to think about, some this will result in a blessed mindset and a bright house.

16.	Be creative; get a new hobby which involves making or creating something – as this will shift your mind's attention, which can bring a better result to an earlier problem.

As you will undoubtedly be looking at
the same problem with a new mindset
and maybe even from a different
angle or viewpoint (mind-opening,
this can be found under meditations
within this book, please take a look)

17.   Exercise – join a health club
and get a regime of how to get fit; this
will not only clean your mind, you
may also enjoy yourself and, of
course, the bonus of losing a few
pounds at the same time.

18.   Be social – as this can open one's mind to new ways of tackling a problem, for instance, thinking of a situation or problem that is bugging you, and then getting others to solve it as a question that you may ask a social event.

19.   Head to a public place; shopping sometimes helps if the shopping list is not too big, haha, However, on the other hand, it does give a person, there personal time to window shop and wonder if they were

to buy something outside of their
normal budge or style, what would
happen.

20.   Pizza night – always a must,
food therapy, with the added cuddles
on the sofa watching something on
the magic talking box (TV), on the
wall.

21.   Sometimes, alcohol can help
within the measure, of course, but the
problems only go away if it is drinking

in moderation. Anything else means you may forget what you managed to figure out the night before about issues or questions you may have had.

22.   Writing to friends can induce stress because we all need someone to talk to who does not talk back sometimes. Sometimes we just need to Babel on about everything and nothing.

23.   Spend time with family,
sometimes someone old or related,
can just make things better.

24.   Forgiveness is the essential
feeling knowing you have no issues or
problems with anyone. Because until
you forgive from your heart, the
burden stays with you epically if
someone has offended you in some
way. Forgive them to their face or
behind their back, makes no
difference, as forgiveness is

forgiveness; it is for you to feel the
power of forgiveness within.

Chap. 17 - Warrior healing,

NEW MUSCLES - after the gym
work out, muscles tend to be saw, and
some of us even try to go that bit far
and end up pulling a muscle - the
cure aside from conventional
medicine, lotions and creams -

Pernation gel – green lipped muscle
extract gel – sooths out pulled
muscles and eases and relaxes saw
and over worked out muscles –
through heating up the affected area,
works wonders and brings new
meaning to the words, wellbeing and
effortlessness.

NEW LEGS - after leg work out at the gym, the veins are entwined with one another, stretching can easy this, however, in some cases the legs can be left feeling tired and saw - vein & leg massage gel is needed thereafter. It brings that sense of relaxing feeling when one is pampering themselves at the spar, this can ease legs and veins, give one that invigorating sensation and smooth out that tired skin and more importantly leave legs feeling lighter. I personally use the one made

by Antitax which can be bought from
Amazon.com (Switzerland).

CASTOR OIL – promotes wound healing, after a session at the gym, morning run or walking put this all over your body. This speed up healing due to its Impressive Anti-Inflammatory Effects of wound healing. This surly is a must, we all need to oil ourselves. After all, this is one of the ways, that solders/warriors would stay healthy by making sure they were well-oiled, then steamed and nourished for the journey that lay ahead.

Step 1. after a shower or bath oil
yourself

Step 2. then rinse off. as the excess
will vanish, leaving a comfy textured
feeling health and wellbeing. After all,
we are warriors in our own way, doing
our own thing.

Eye muscle strain movements

ERM radiation effects some of us, as
we are spending more and more time
in front of electronics devises; from
these devises is where we collect that

negative eons from and feel the

fatigue and strain of eyes, headaches

and neck muscles, because we are

exposed to invisible radiation which

brings us down quite somewhat.

<u>The first cure</u>

This an ancient eye technique
which was taught to our family
by their grandparents, by
using the palms of your
hands,

Step 1. Rub your palms
together really fast, so you can
feel your palms heating up.

Step 2. Close your eyes,
firmly, like you are going to
sleep.

Step 3. Place your palms over
your eyes for 10 seconds and
let go.

Step 4. Keep your eyes closed

Step 5. Try these three times.

The energy that your hands
are bringing together very fast
is curing your eyes and the
heat part of the process
warms up the muscles around
your eyes.

<u>The second cure</u>

This 5-minute meditations, please put
any sound or meditation on for this
process.

> Step 1. Rub your palms
> together really fast, so you can
> feel your palms heating up.

> Step 2. Close your eyes,
> firmly, like you are going to
> sleep.

Step 3. Place your palms over
your eyes for 10 seconds and
let go.

Step 4. Keep your eyes
closed.

Step 5. Lay down somewhere
comfortable.

Step 6. Place a slice of
cucumber on each eye.

Step 7. As the cucumber starts
to sink its minerals over your
eyes.

Step 8. Try to tear out, (cry)
the salt tears will interact with
the minerals.

Step 9. After 5 min.

Step 10. Wake up and wash
your face with warm water.

<u>The Third cure</u>

Take pictures with your eyes
by blinking as a camera shutter
would,

Step 1. Move your eyes to the
left. (only eyeballs).

Step 2. Move your eyes to the
right. (only eyeballs)

Step 3. Move your eyes to the
up. (only eyeballs).

Step 4. Move your eyes to the

down. (only eyeballs)

Step 5. Try these three times.

Step 6. Then take a mental

picture of something dark.

Step 7. Then take a mental

picture of something light.

Step 8. Then take a mental
picture of five objects of
different colour.

Step 9. After 3 min.

Step 10. Blink really fast,

Step 11. Blink really slow,
(slowly closing the eye lids).

Step 12. Wash your face with
cold water and feel refreshed.

<u>The fourth cure</u>

Stand in any room, which is blacked
out, (very dark).

> Step 1. Rub index and middle
> fingers together really fast.

> Step 2. Close your eyes, tight,
> (like something dreadful is
> going to happen).

Step 3. Place your fingers over
your eyes for 20 seconds and
let go.

Step 4. And then quickly
open your eyes.

Step 5. Look around & you
should be able to see shadows
of objects within the room.

Step 6. This will reset your
eyes.

Step 7. After 3 minutes come
out of the room or put the
light on.

Step 8. Wash your face with
warm water.

<u>The fifth cure</u>

Stand in any room and look at your index fingers of any hand.

> Step 1. Put your hand right in front of you,

> Step 2. Make a fist and hold out your index finger,

> Step 3. Move the finger left to right slowly, (do not move your head).

Step 5. Step 4. Follow your
finger with your eyeballs (do
not blink).

Step 6. Do this for 20
seconds, and then stop.

Step 7. Take a rest and try
this process for three times.

Step 8. Then look at
something 10 – 20 feet away.

Step 9. However, this time
move your head but not your
eye balls.

Step 10. And move your head
side to side whilst keeping
your eyes focused on the item
in the room, which you have
choose to focus on.

Step 11. Do this for 20
seconds, and then stop.

Step 12. Take a rest and try
this process for three times.

This should reset the coordination
within your eyes, and hopefully ease
the strain of everyday life.

<u>The sixth cure</u>

The next cure is one of practise at
work, and not one from the oldies.

1. Reduce the
   thermostat.

2. Take regular breaks.

3. Reduce light on
   monitors, tv etc.

4. Use a humidifier.

5. Use a aroma oil
    diffuser.

6. Change your glasses
    or eye wear.

7. Quite smoking.

8. Hold your eye lids
    shut for 20 – 30
    seconds and release.

9. Lower contrast on any
    devise.

10. Take nature walks

11. Try the 20-20-20 rule
    – every 20 minutes
    look at something 20
    feet away for 20
    seconds.

12. Change the air in the
    room, (open a
    window).

CAYENNE PEPPER AND OLIVE OIL – used to heal that twitch on your knee; that bump on the funny bone and heal small arthritis related issues, (Canada).

PAAYA CURRY, - Commonly known as the Indian version of broth. This soup curry has the healing power to heal fractured bones heal. It has the magic to strengthen bones when they are weak, (Central Asia).

PERNATION GEL – ease those stiff

joints, no longer do we need to rely

on pain killers to ease that cold

winters aches, there is a remedy

created, a simple massage into the

skin, works wonders, (Switzerland).

211

FOOT CARE CREAM – we walk on them; they help us so much; we can't do without them; some of us forget the part our feet play in our lives. Stop and pamper them once every month, if not every week, why wait for them to stop you in your tracks? Act now and apply the Swedish formula on your feet; believe me when I say it feels like a slice of heaven. Take time out of your day to do something that will benefit you tremendously, (Sweden).

ROTI (CHAPATI) HEALING –

This is an ancient healing technique, used when there is either muscle tension in the legs or there is a rash of some sort. Soon as the roti is made, olive oil is brushed on and the roti is then tied to the leg and as the heat compressions works, the oil reacts to the wound effectively.

IMMUNE SYSTEM CLEANSE –
consume two tablespoons of seven
seas cod liver oil, which is high in
omega 3 nutrients. One of the most
important is vitamin D, which cod
liver oil is rich in. I remember, as a
child, this was compulsory to have. At
the time, I hated it, now I thank my
parents for the excellent immune
system that I bear as a result. To the
age of the social media, such things
get overlooked and I guess in many
ways that's what this book is all about.
Can help during Autumn and winter

when the sun cannot provide the

vitamin D as much as it can in the

spring and summer.

<u>Anti-ageing healing,</u>

AGELESS SKIN – natural youth skin, how you ask!!! Well; collagen promotes health skin according to leading scientists in the field of antiaging. Of course, some people believe collagen to be an ingredient of a face lotion. What if I said collagen can be consumed too? It is crazy, but yes, you can buy a multi collagen powder containing all the goodness of a cream in a powder that can be consumed by adding it into your

morning tea or coffee; and scatter it
over your morning porridge. Yes, it is
that simple. Eat and drink your way
to heathier skin.

AGELESS FACE – Retinol, more commonly known as vitamin A. which starts to decline in your 30s. This needs to be replaced through expensive creams. Really, No, No, No, look on Amazon.com and see for yourself, the creams are a fraction of the price. Just remember to use the ones that have 2.5% retinol and above. Let's look and feel good united.

AGELESS Look – lemon juice, drink
this were possible and add into
mixtures and foods alike as it is an
antitoxin. It cures most things; to
point out just a few, swine flu, cold,
kidney stones, and even ringing in the
ears. It is also high in vitamin C,
which helps protect the immune
system, so the immune system can
help defend against illness against
your wellbeing. And help with weight
loss too.

EGCG – helps battle wrinkles and helps cell increase turnover (China).

Conclusion,

Rather than give your opinion or review, please take a moment and think, what may not work for you, may work for someone else. This book is a bout healing, so, please refrain from giving bad review's, because someone just may discourage themselves from something which may have done wonders for them. By reading a bad review from someone that may have not either misunderstood something or may be

being unkind because the method
didn't work for them.

If something doesn't work, please try
something else. After all, any medical
practitioner will only do just that,
before finding the right treatment for
you. That is what this book is all
about, finding what works best for
you.

Children of the future need to know
of the past remedies because
otherwise how will they build on the

legacies of the past. Passing down the knowledge is human forte, sometimes the previous remedies may be more effective than the modern medicines. It is our job to provide the information for the youngsters of tomorrow so they can have a guideline to obtain natural extracts. That's what we are doing, we are merely compiling ancient forgotten remedies which tomorrows people can look upon after we are not here one day.

Behind the healing,

Behind the healing,

Disclaimer: The information here is not medical advice; we advise that you consult a physician before beginning any herbal tea therapy.

Disclaimer: The information here is not medical advice; we advise that you consult a physician before beginning any juice therapy.

Disclaimer: The information here is
not medical advice; we advise that
you consult a physician before
beginning any herbal therapy.

Disclaimer: The information here is
not medical advice; we advise that
you consult a physician before
beginning any muscle therapy.

Disclaimer: The information here is
not medical advice or beautician
based; we advise that you consult a
physician or a beautician before

beginning any beauty wellbeing and facial treatment.

Disclaimer: The information here is not medical advice; we advise that you consult a physician before beginning any antiaging treatment(s).

Disclaimer: The information here is not medical advice; we advise that you consult a physician before beginning any aroma oil(s), treatment(s).

Disclaimer: The information is not a
monk or guru related; we advise that
you consult a spiritual practitioner
before beginning any mental
enlightenment treatment(s).

Disclaimer: The information is based
on personal experience; we advise
that you consult a spiritual
practitioner before beginning any
mental enlightenment treatment(s).

Disclaimer: The information here is
based on personal theories that are

researched through one's own experiences. I believe they work based on my exploits alone and what I have learned in my travels from people who have taught me inside into forgiveness; we advise that you consult a spiritual practitioner before beginning any mental enlightenment treatment(s).

www.ingramcontent.com/pod-product-compliance
Lightning Source LLC
Chambersburg PA
CBHW031100250726
48655CB00004B/1523